Calico Cat's Exercise Book

written and illustrated by Donald Charles

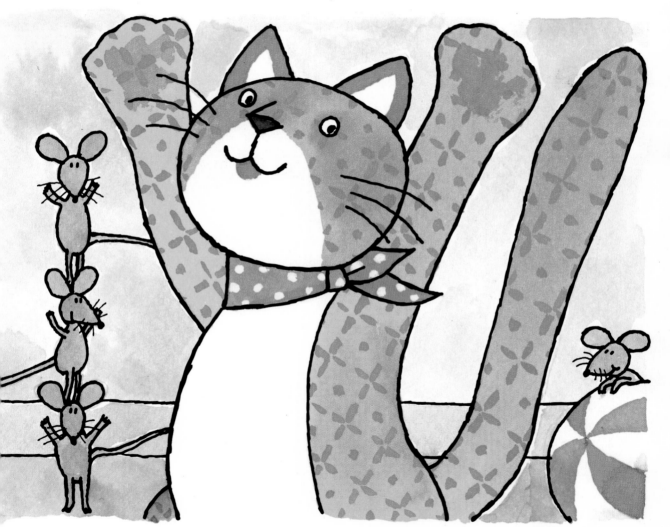

CHILDRENS PRESS, CHICAGO

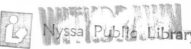

E

for Cristina and Brandon

Library of Congress Cataloging in Publication Data

Charles, Donald.
  Calico cat's exercise book.

  Summary: Calico Cat demonstrates various
exercises to his class of mice.
  [1. Exercise—Fiction. 2. Cats—Fiction]
I. Title.
PZ7.C374Cam   1982   [E]   82-9640
ISBN 0-516-03457-X

Calico Cat's Exercise Book

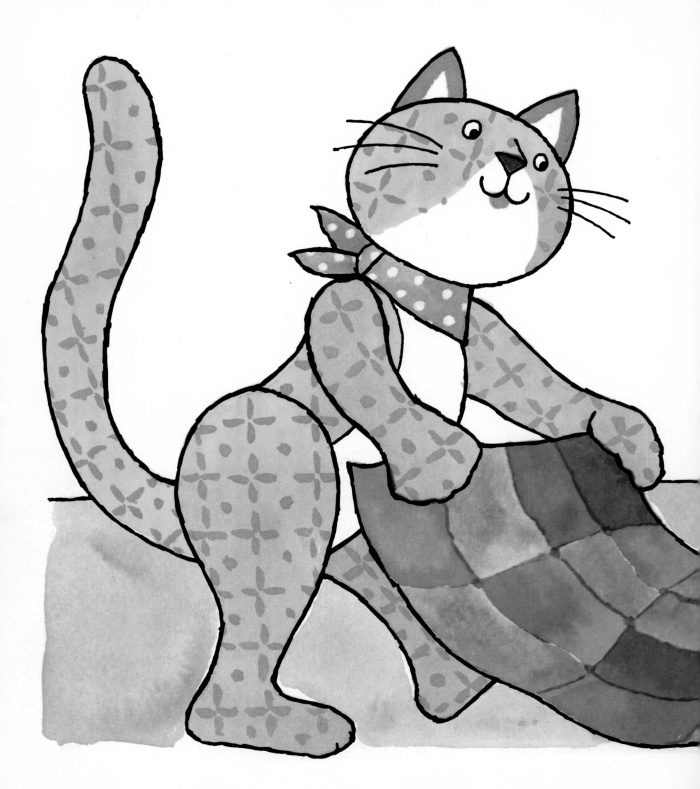

Calico Cat
likes to exercise
every day.

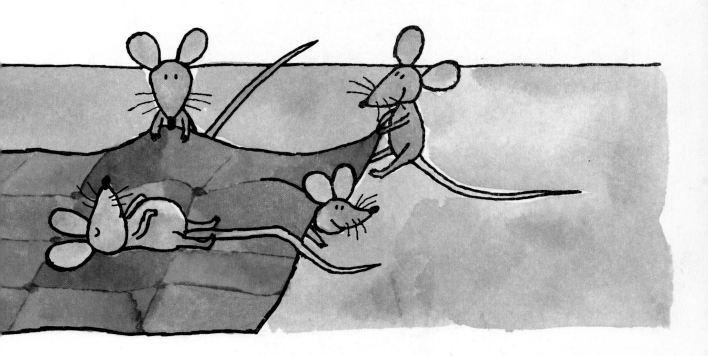

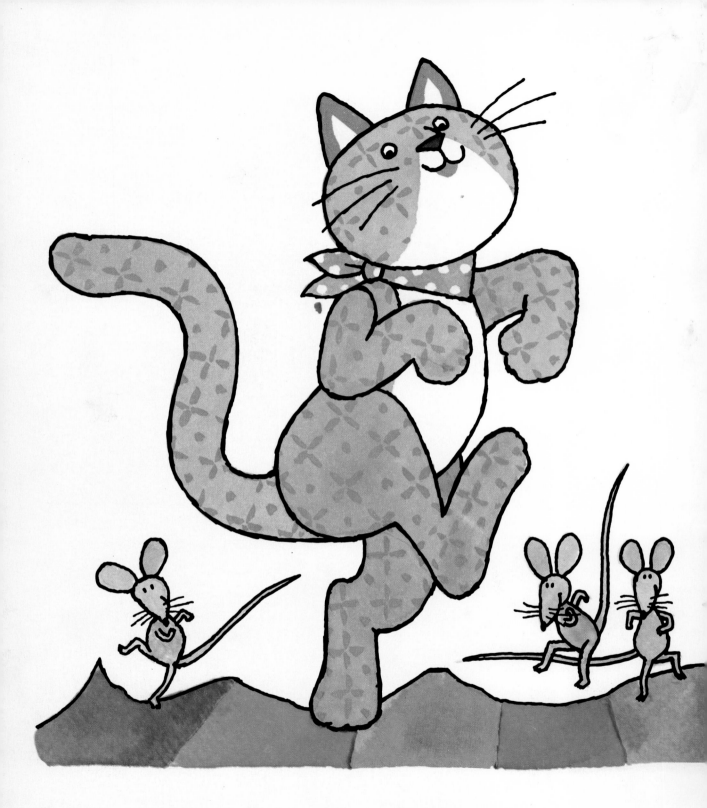

Run in place.
Jog, jog, jog.

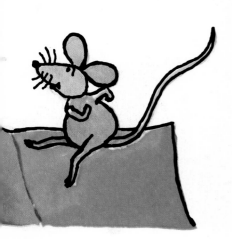

One, two, one, two:
Jumping jacks.

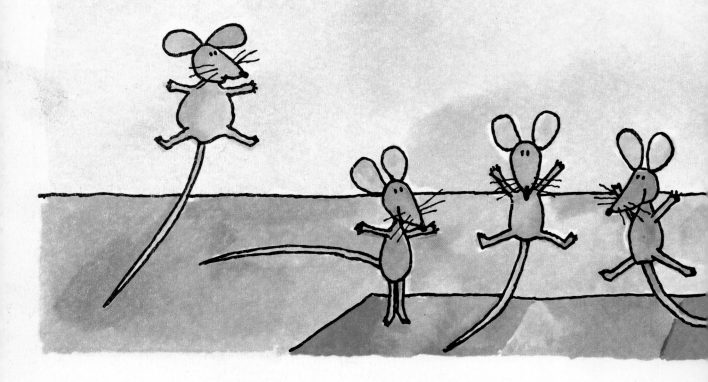

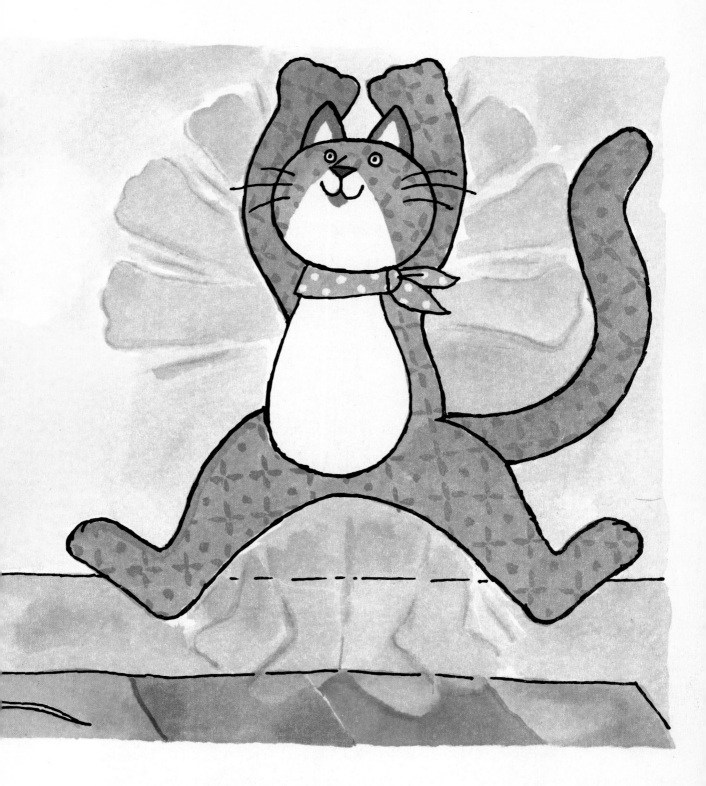

9

Skip rope.

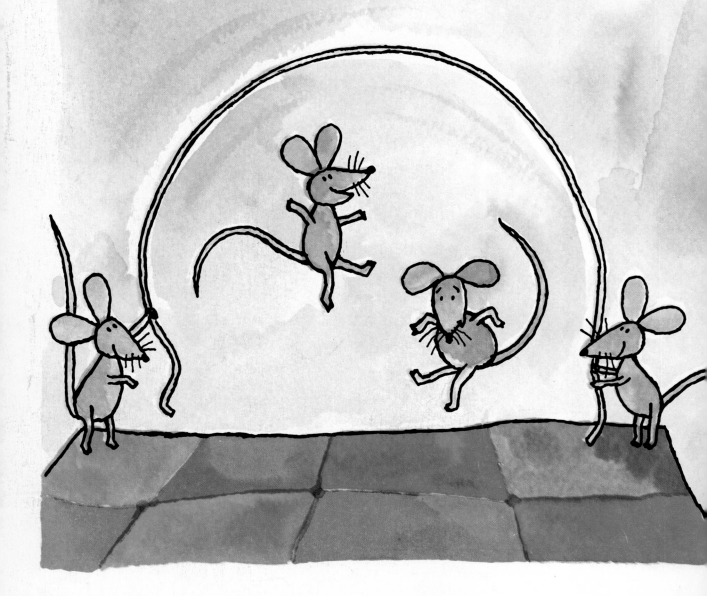

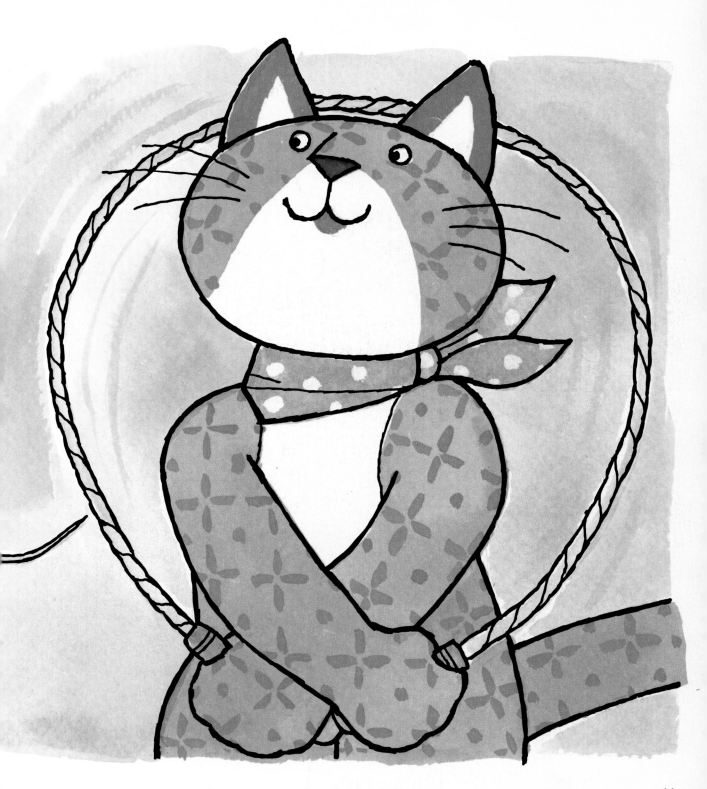

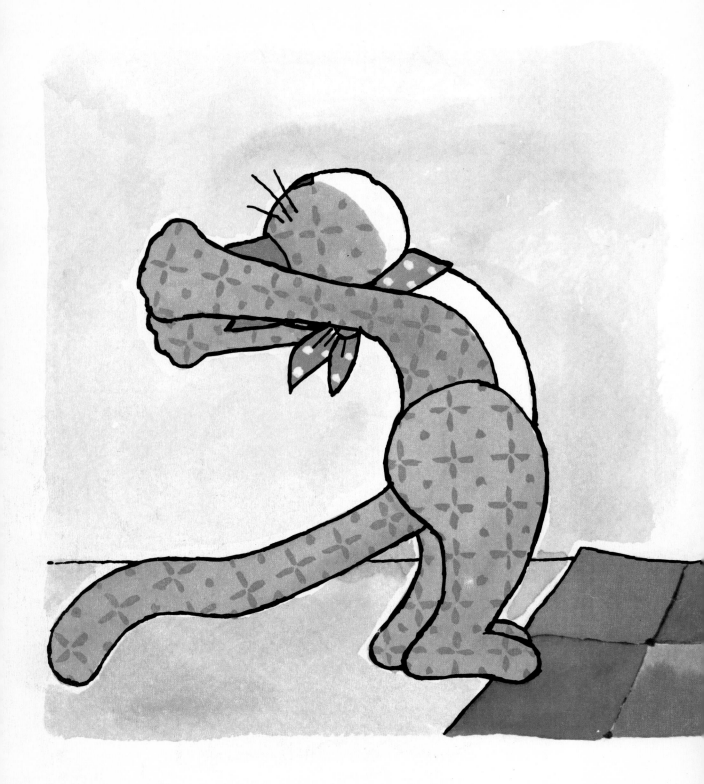

Bend and stretch.

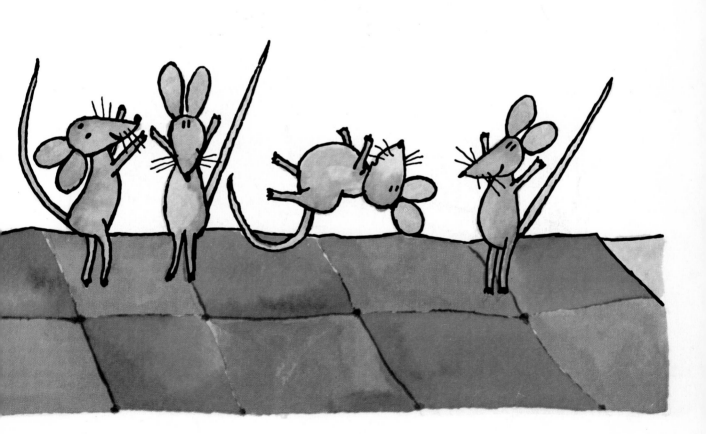

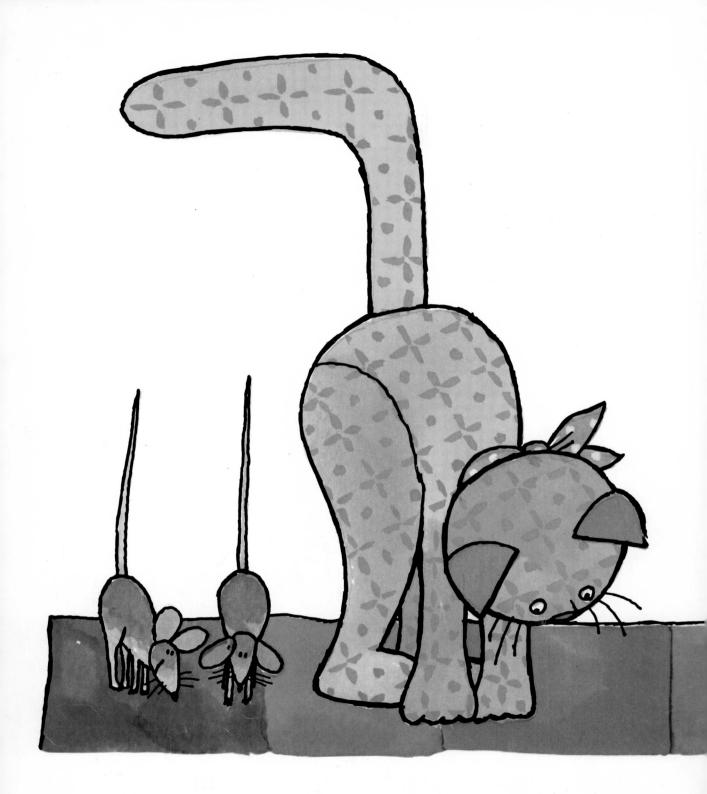

Touch your toes.

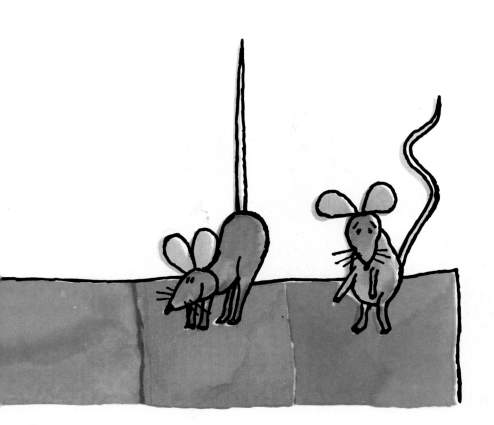

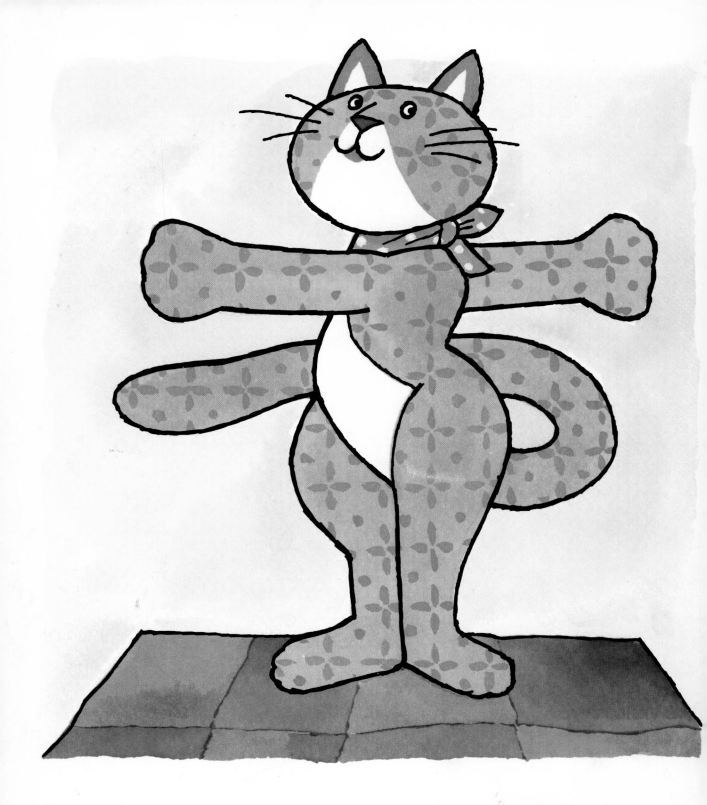

Twist left.
Twist right.

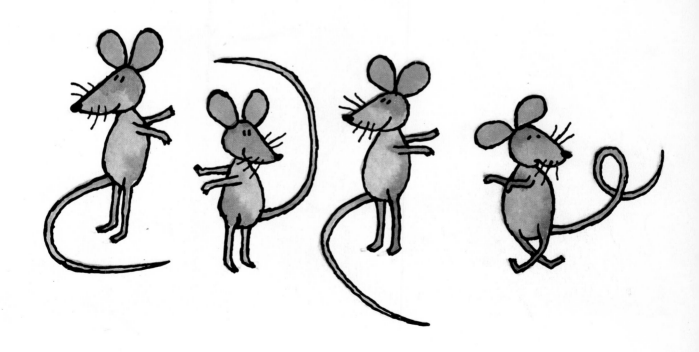

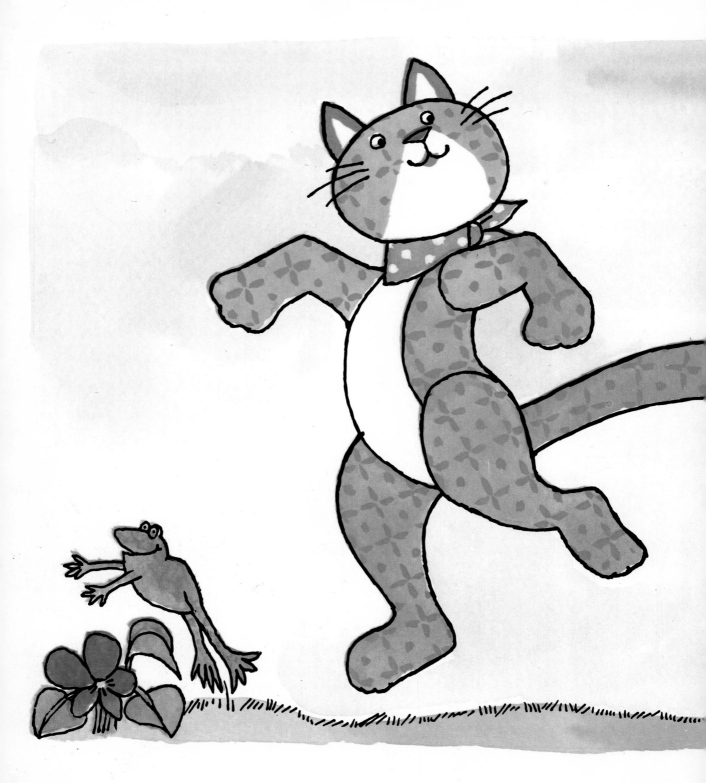

Hop, hop.

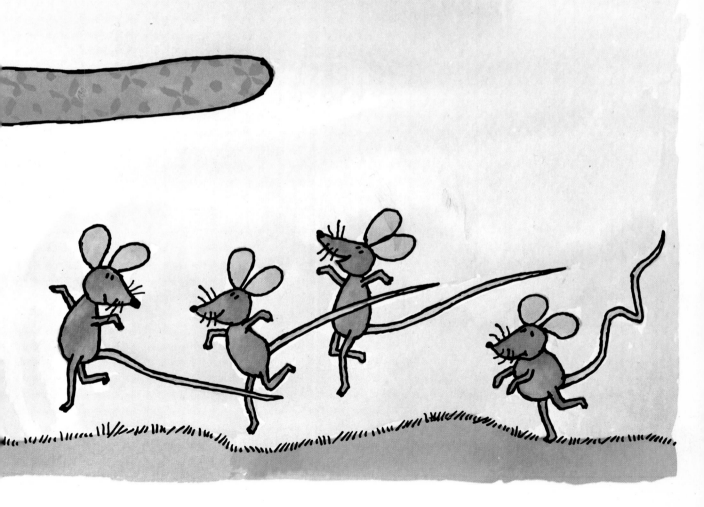

Roll right.
Roll left.

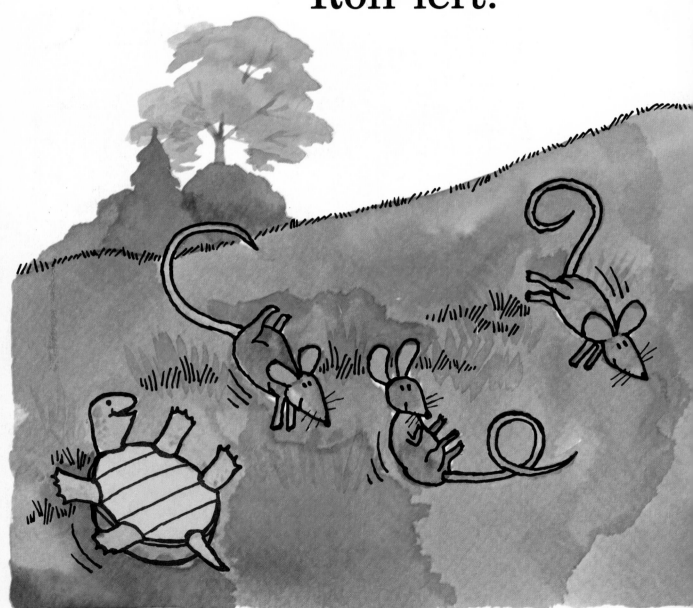

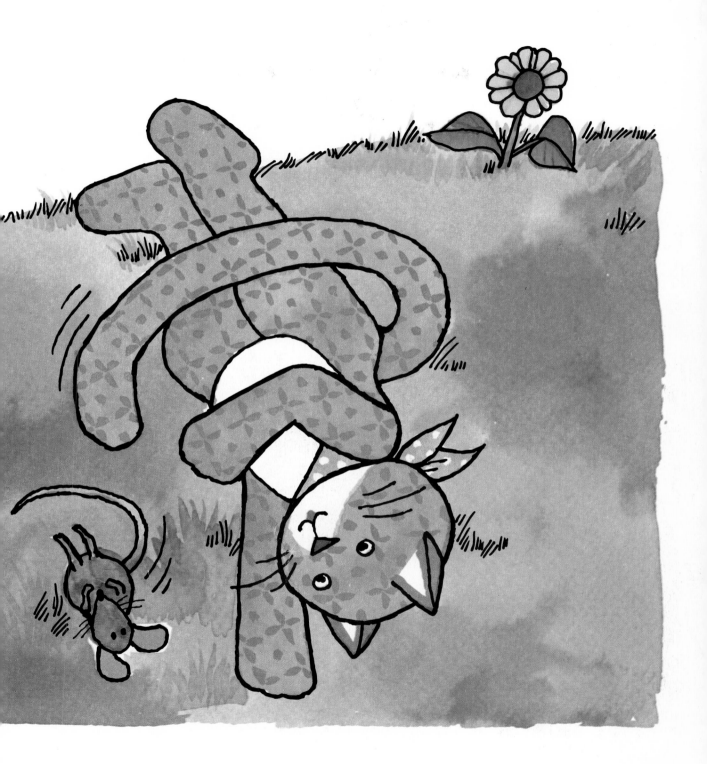

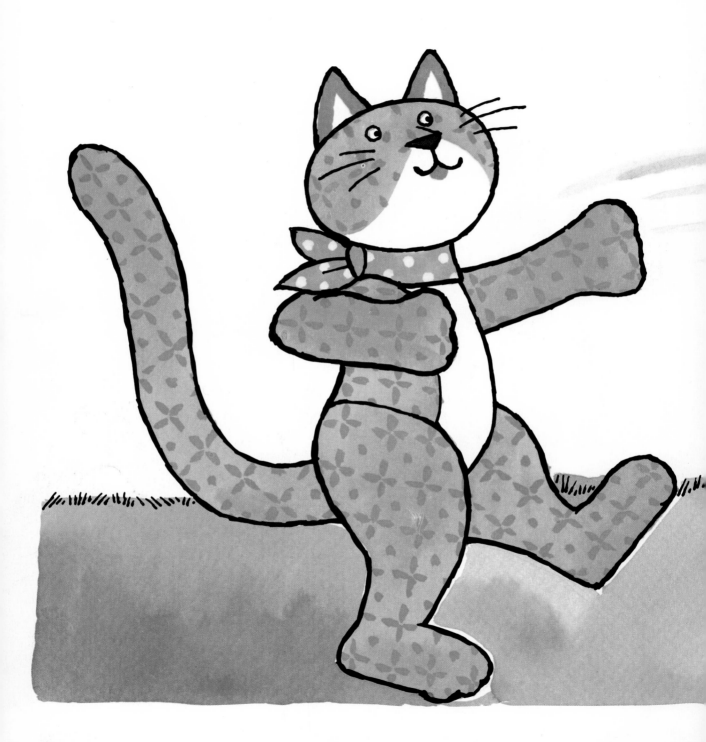

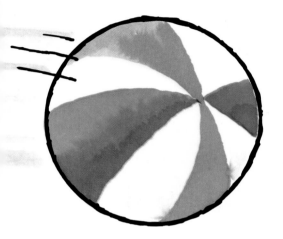

Throw.

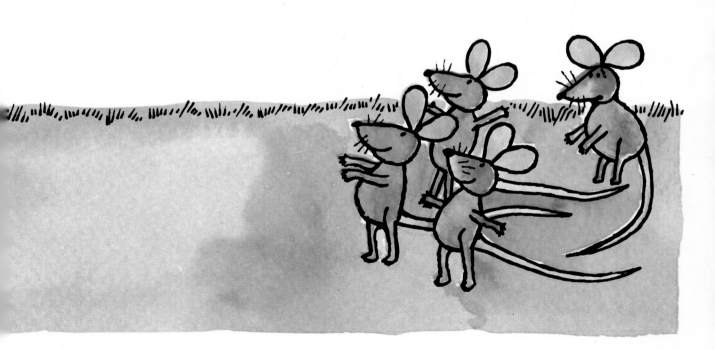

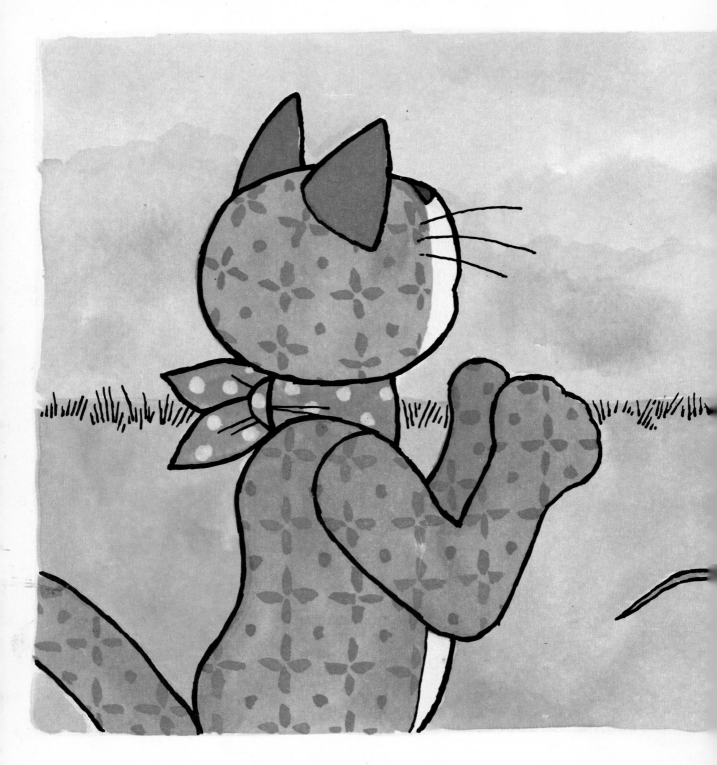

Catch.

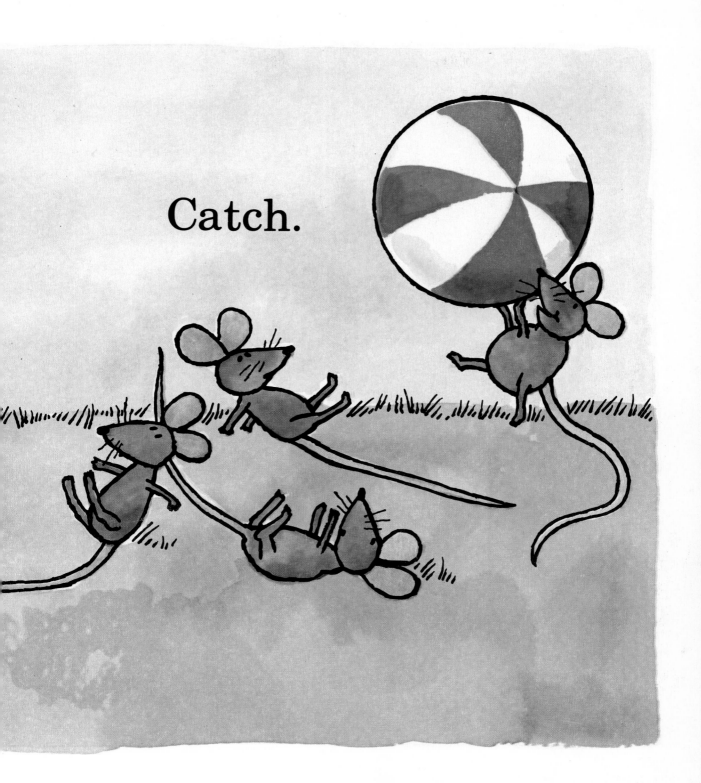

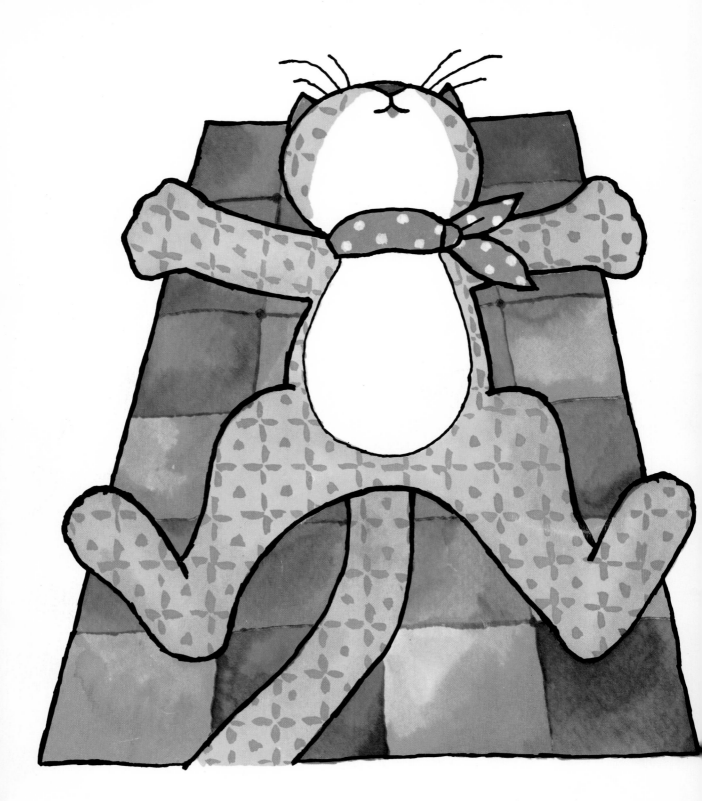

Rest.

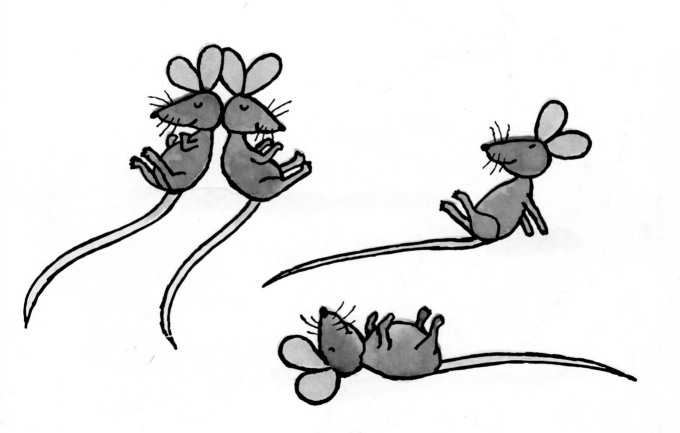

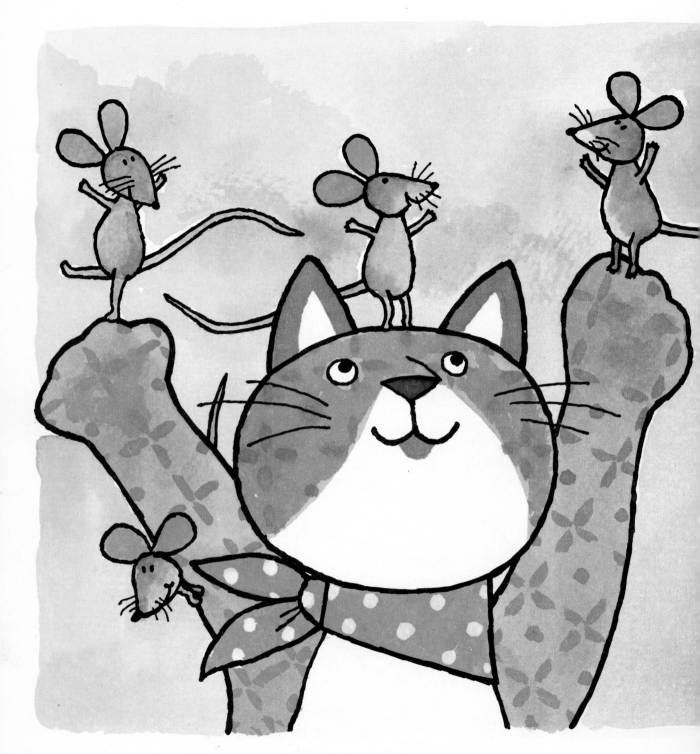

Calico Cat
feels fit
and trim.

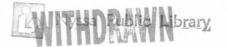

Calico Cat can
do exercises.
Can you?

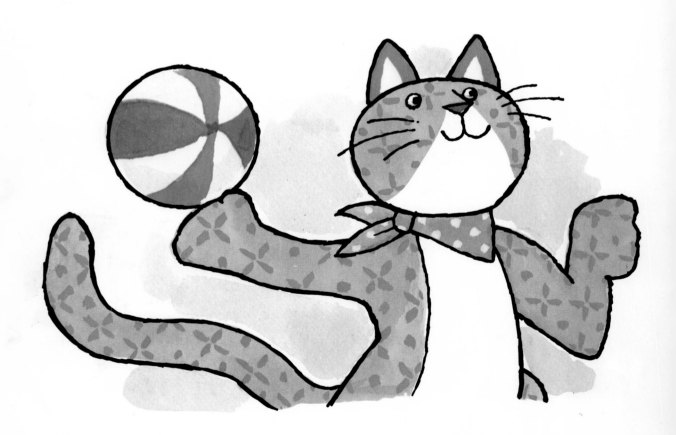

Run
Jump
Skip
Bend
Stretch
Touch toes
Twist
Hop
Roll
Throw
Catch

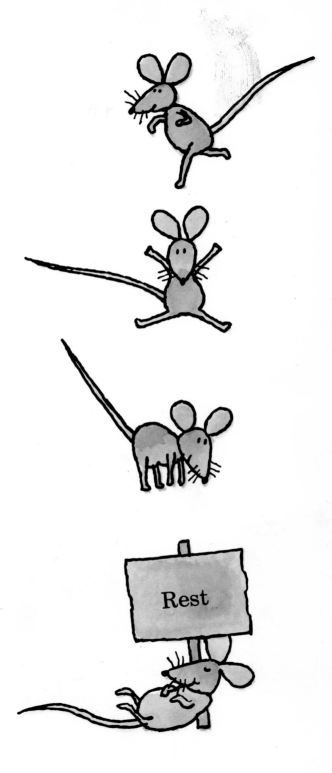

Rest

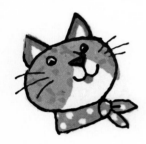

ABOUT THE AUTHOR/ARTIST

Donald Charles started his long career as an artist and author more than twenty-five years ago after attending the University of California and the Art League School of California. He began by writing and illustrating feature articles for the *San Francisco Chronicle,* and also sold cartoons and ideas to *The New Yorker* and *Cosmopolitan* magazines. Since then he has been, at various times, a longshoreman, ranch hand, truck driver, and editor of a weekly newspaper, all enriching experiences for a writer and artist. Ultimately he became creative director for an advertising agency, a post which he resigned several years ago to devote himself full-time to book illustration and writing. Mr. Charles has received frequent awards from graphic societies, and his work has appeared in numerous textbooks and periodicals.